Nursing & Health Survival Guide

Patient Consent

Elizabeth Charnock and Denise Owens

T0186504

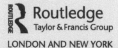

Routledge
Taylor & Francis Group

LONDON AND NEW YORK

First published 2014
by Routledge
2 Park Square, Milton Park, Abingdon, Oxon, OX14 4RN

and by Routledge
711 Third Avenue, New York, NY10017

Routledge is an imprint of the Taylor & Francis Group, an informa business

British Library Cataloguing in Publication Data
A catalogue record for this book is available from the British Library

Library of Congress Cataloging in Publication Data
A catalog record has been requested for this book

ISBN: 978-0-273-77517-1 (pbk)
ISBN: 978-0-273-77519-5 (ebk)

Typeset in 8/9.5pt Helvetica by Graphicraft Limited, Hong Kong

contents

Patient consent: a significant contribution to respectful patient care

Patient consent to treatment is a legal and ethical requirement. Professional codes and standards, produced by regulatory bodies to guide clinical practice, highlight patient consent as being fundamental to professional and compassionate care (Health and Care Professions Council, 2012; General Medical Council, 2008; Nursing and Midwifery Council, 2008). Gaining patient consent prior to medical/nursing examinations or treatments is not an optional extra set aside for consideration by only the more conscientious practitioners, nor is it only to be reserved for treatments considered to carry a risk to the patient's safety. It is essential for healthcare practitioners to gain patient consent prior to any treatment that involves touching the patient. In the case of the patient who lacks the capacity to consent, the practitioner must be able to justify the treatment as being lawful and in the best interests of the patient.

The 6 Cs (care, compassion, competence, communication, courage and commitment), the values deemed essential to the provision of respectful and compassionate care (Department of Health, 2012), are fundamental to the process of consent. The process of consent is one that demands: the practitioner's **care** and **commitment** to treatment that respects the right of the autonomous patient to determine what happens to them; the **compassion** and **communication** skills to engage the patient in meaningful and sensitive discussions about their treatment; the **courage** to advocate on behalf of the patient to ensure that the process of consent is duly considered within the multiprofessional partnership of care; and the **competence** to contribute to the process of consent and treatment decisions made in the best interests of the patient who lacks the capacity to consent.

Underlying principles of patient consent

■ THE IMPORTANCE OF PATIENT CONSENT

In the light of the inquiry into the care of children at the Bristol Royal Infirmary, the Kennedy Report (Bristol Royal Infirmary Inquiry, 2001) stressed the importance of gaining patient consent prior to *any* treatments or clinical procedures that involve touching the patient and not just those, such as surgical interventions, considered to pose a high risk to patient safety. The recommendations emphasise that gaining consent is much more than a 'one-off' task of obtaining a signature on a form; it is instead a process of informing and communicating effectively with the patient and, if appropriate, their family.

- In the absence of a real or valid consent to treatment, or alternative legal justification for the treatment, a claim of trespass to the person could result.
- In suing for trespass to the person, the claim is one of battery (actually touching the patient without their consent or alternative legal justification) and/or assault (where the patient was in fear of being touched against their wishes).

(Dimond, 2011)

■ WHO SHOULD GAIN PATIENT CONSENT?

- The practitioner who is going to carry out the investigation or treatment does not necessarily need to be the one who obtains the patient's consent – this can be delegated to another appropriately trained and competent practitioner.
- It is, however, the responsibility of the practitioner carrying out the investigation or treatment to ensure that a valid patient consent has been obtained.

- The practitioner who gains the consent needs to be knowledgeable about the proposed treatment or investigation to give accurate information to the patient and respond to all the patient's questions and concerns.
- All practitioners need to be aware of their limitations and are responsible for seeking help from more experienced and knowledgeable colleagues if they are unsure in any part of the process of gaining consent.

(Department of Health, 2009)

■ VERBAL CONSENT

Healthcare practitioners owe a duty of care to the patient to ensure that consent is gained prior to *any* treatment or clinical procedure that involves touching the patient. Not all treatments and procedures will, however, require written consent; in certain circumstances, verbal or implied forms of consent will suffice.

Verbal consent to treatment is agreed through discussion and negotiation with the patient and is a feature of general everyday care activity and treatments considered to pose less risk to patients (Dimond, 2011).

- Discussing care and proposed treatments with patients should not be viewed by practitioners as an inconvenience but instead as an essential component of everyday practice and a prerequisite to building a therapeutic partnership built on trust.

■ IMPLIED CONSENT

In implied consent, the patient demonstrates clearly via non-verbal language that they consent to the treatment being offered; for example, by lifting their top to allow for and facilitate the auscultation of their chest or by lifting their shirt sleeve, revealing and positioning their arm to facilitate venepuncture, or, in the case of a parent, assisting in positioning and holding still their young child's head to facilitate an aural examination.

- The problem with implied consent is that the treatment usually occurs with little or no negotiation or information being relayed to the patient about the treatment.
- An assumption is made by the practitioner that the patient understands the treatment offered but the risk is that they may not. If a patient does not understand the treatment or why they are having the treatment, consent is invalid.
- To avoid the practitioner incorrectly assuming that the patient understands and agrees to the proposed treatment, practitioners are advised to inform the patient about what they intend to do and seek their verbal agreement prior to performing the treatment.

(Dimond, 2011)

■ WRITTEN CONSENT

Written consent involves the patient signing a consent form to confirm that they agree to the proposed treatment. Although written patient consent is not generally a legal requirement (other than under specific terms of the Mental Health Act 1983 and the Human Fertilisation and Embryology Act 2008), it is considered good practice to obtain written consent prior to the patient undergoing surgery (Department of Health, 2009). The Department of Health (2009), as part of their review of the *Reference Guide to Consent for Examination or Treatment*, offer advice regarding the content of a range of consent forms to reflect the requirements of the

Mental Capacity Act 2005 and influential case law regarding the requirements of a valid consent. The consent form used should reflect the specific needs of the patient with regard to consent; for example:

- Adults and young people over 16 years who have the capacity to consent for treatment.
- Consent from a person with parental responsibility on behalf of a child.
- Consent for procedures that do not impair consciousness.
- In cases where the adult lacks the capacity to consent to treatment, the decision, based on the best interests of the patient, should be justified in writing (Department of Health, 2009).

Obtaining written patient consent involves much more than completing the task of gaining the patient's signature on a form. Gaining patient consent is a process of informing and communicating with the patient to check their understanding of the proposed treatment and their willingness to consent.

- Written consent should, if possible and appropriate, be gained well in advance of the proposed treatment, therefore giving the patient time to discuss, question and fully consider the proposed treatment.
- When written consent has been gained in advance of the treatment, practitioners need to check with the patient that they still consent at the time of the treatment.

(Department of Health, 2009)

■ THE MENTAL CAPACITY ACT 2005

The Mental Capacity Act 2005 applies to people aged 16 and over. The Act provides a statutory framework, based on five key principles, to empower and protect vulnerable people who are not able to make their own decisions (Box 1).

- The Act makes it clear who can take decisions, in which situations, and how they should go about this. It enables people to plan ahead for a time when they may lose capacity.
- The Mental Capacity Act 2005 replaces previous statutory schemes for Enduring Powers of Attorney and Court of Protection Receivers with reformed and updated schemes.

Box 1
The Mental Capacity Act 2005 Section 1

The principles
1. The following principles apply for the purposes of this Act.
2. A person must be assumed to have capacity unless it is established that he lacks capacity.
3. A person is not to be treated as unable to make a decision unless all practicable steps to help him to do so have been taken without success.
4. A person is not to be treated as unable to make a decision merely because he makes an unwise decision.
5. An act done, or decision made, under this Act for or on behalf of a person who lacks capacity must be done, or made, in his best interests.
6. Before the act is done, or the decision is made, regard must be had to whether the purpose for which it is needed can be as effectively achieved in a way that is less restrictive of the person's rights and freedom of action.

Source: http://www.legislation.gov.uk

- The Act aims to empower people who lack capacity to remain at the centre of the decision-making process and to safeguard them and the professionals who work with them.

■ THE REQUIREMENTS OF A VALID CONSENT

For consent to be valid, three requirements must be met. The patient or proxy/person with parental responsibility (as in the case of children who lack the capacity to consent) must:

1. Give consent voluntarily.
2. Receive relevant and adequate information to inform the decision.
3. Have the capacity to make the required decision.

■ VOLUNTARINESS

The patient or proxy (person with parental responsibility) must give their consent to treatment freely without undue influence or pressure from anyone else. It is up to the patient or person with parental responsibility to decide whether to give consent to treatment or not. The patient, by merit of their illness, discomfort, pain or fear, may be particularly vulnerable to the powerful influence of others.

- Family members, parents and members of the multidisciplinary team all have the potential to exert undue pressure on the patient regarding a treatment decision.
- When possible, speaking to the patient on their own, away from the influence of family members, provides an opportunity for practitioners to gauge the real wishes of the patient.

- Practitioners should avoid expressing personal opinions and ethical views about treatment to patients as this may put undue pressure on the patient to comply with the views expressed.

(Department of Health, 2009; Hendrick, 2010)

■ RELEVANT INFORMATION

The process of gaining consent includes sharing and discussing information with the patient or person with parental responsibility. The information discussed with patients should take into account the individual patient's needs or wishes, and their level of knowledge and understanding, and should be proportionate to their condition and the complexity and risk of the proposed treatment (General Medical Council, 2008).

- To give consent to treatment, the patient, or the person with parental responsibility, requires relevant information based on what they both *need and want to know* about the proposed treatment, such as (the following is not an exhaustive list):
  - The patient's condition, prognosis and all available treatment options.
  - The purpose of the proposed treatment and an explanation of what it involves.
  - The potential consequences of not performing the treatment.
  - The potential benefits, success rates, risks and burdens of the treatment proposed.
  - Whether the proposed treatment is part of a research study.
  - The patient's right to refuse consent and to seek a second opinion (General Medical Council, 2008).

- Some patients may not want detailed information about the proposed treatment or investigation and, as far as possible, their wishes should be respected. In such instances, every effort must be made to ascertain and, if possible, remedy, why the patient does not want to discuss the proposed treatment. However, to gain the patient's consent, it is necessary that the patient receives enough information regarding the nature and purpose of the treatment to inform their decision (Department of Health, 2009).
- It may become apparent that the patient does not understand what they have given consent for, so rendering the consent invalid (e.g. the patient may have signed a consent form but later asks 'What did I just sign?'). In such instances, practitioners have a legal duty of care to the patient to ensure that the person responsible for gaining the consent resumes discussion with the patient. Further discussion with the patient will need to relay relevant information to aid the patient's understanding and confirm their consent (Dimond, 2011).
- A claim of negligence could result if the patient's consent is not informed adequately by information pertinent to the treatment decision (Hendrick, 2010).

■ THE IMPORTANCE OF GOOD COMMUNICATION

The Mental Capacity Act 2005 emphasises the importance of helping people to make their own decisions.
- Information should be relayed to the patient in a way that is appropriate to their needs to put them at ease and aid their understanding. Non-verbal communication, visual

aids, simplistic language or interpreter services may be required.
(Department for Constitutional Affairs, 2007)

■ CAPACITY

In the legal context, mental capacity is the ability to make decisions (British Medical Association, 2008a). Examples of the situations in which it might be particularly important to establish a person's mental capacity include when making choices and decisions about finances or undertaking or making a will or Lasting Power of Attorney. Establishing mental capacity or incapacity might also be particularly important in relation to decisions about an individual's physical wellbeing and about medical treatment that he or she may require now or in the future (Department for Constitutional Affairs, 2007, Chapter 4).

To give consent, the patient or the person with parental responsibility must have the capacity, or in other words be competent, to make the required decision.

- Unlike children, adults and young people aged 16–17 years are presumed to have the capacity/ competence to consent to medical treatment unless there is evidence to prove otherwise.

For adults and young people aged 16–17 years old, Sections 2 and 3 of the Mental Capacity Act 2005 guide the assessment of capacity, which is in two stages (see Boxes 2 and 3).

People are considered to lack capacity if they have an impairment that causes them to be unable to make a specific decision (Box 2).

Box 2
The Mental Capacity Act 2005 Section 2 (1)

People who lack capacity
(1) For the purposes of this Act, a person lacks capacity in relation to a matter if at the material time he is unable to make a decision for himself in relation to the matter because of an impairment of, or a disturbance in the functioning of, the mind or brain.

Source: http://www.legislation.gov.uk

- Conditions and circumstances that may impair the patient's ability to make a decision are wide-ranging and include dementia, acute confusion, mental health problems, learning disabilities, substance misuse and distress or emotional disturbance. However, no specific diagnosis should be assumed to imply incapacity. No one can be labelled 'incapable' merely as a result of a particular medical condition or diagnosis (General Medical Council, 2008).

The person giving consent should be able to understand, retain and weigh the information provided and communicate their decision (Box 3).
- Competence requires not only cognitive function, but also the ability to process information in a meaningful way.
- The assessment of mental capacity is specific and applies to each individual decision at any particular time. A new treatment decision will require the practitioner to once

---

Box 3
The Mental Capacity Act 2005 Section 3 (1)

Inability to make decisions
1. For the purposes of Section 2, a person is unable to make a decision for himself if he is unable—
   a. to understand the information relevant to the decision,
   b. to retain that information,
   c. to use or weigh that information as part of the process of making the decision, or
   d. to communicate his decision (whether by talking, using sign language or any other means).

Source: http://www.legislation.gov.uk

---

more consider the patient's capacity to consent. Patients may have the capacity to consent to some but not other treatment decisions.
- Assessment of capacity should not be prejudiced by the person's age, appearance, medical condition or behaviour.

■ THE PRINCIPLE OF NECESSITY IN AN EMERGENCY SITUATION

In an emergency situation, administration of treatment to the *adult* patient who lacks the capacity to consent, in the absence of any knowledge regarding the patient's own wishes regarding such situations, is justifiable as long as the treatment given is vital to the health or survival of the patient (Brazier and Cave, 2007).

In the emergency situation, it is also justifiable to treat the *child* in the absence of consent from a proxy (person with parental responsibility) as long as the treatment is vital to prevent the deterioration of the child's health or is in itself life-saving (Department of Health, 2009).

- In such instances, the defence to treatment is that the urgency of the situation and risk to the health and life of the patient necessitated immediate action and there was no time to wait to gain consent.
- The defence of necessity does not extend to treatment beyond the immediate emergency situation.

Consent and the adult patient

■ RESPECTING THE ADULT PATIENT'S COMPETENT DECISION TO REFUSE TREATMENT

Consent is closely allied to the ethical principle of autonomy, which is the patient's right to determine what happens to them. To be able to make an autonomous decision, the patient must have the capacity to do so. Practitioners do not have to agree with the adult's decision for it to be valid. An adult patient is at liberty to make what others may judge to be an 'unwise' or 'irrational' decision just as long as the patient is competent to do so and therefore fully understands the consequences of their decision (Department of Health, 2009). An example may be where a patient with capacity who has cancer, after receiving and discussing all the relevant information, refuses curative treatment.

- It is important that practitioners do not consider a patient to be incompetent to make their own decisions simply because they do not agree with their views or decisions.

- No one can consent on behalf of a competent adult patient.
- The decision of a competent adult patient, if it fulfils the requirement of a valid consent, must be respected even if this results in their death *except* in specific situations outlined in the Mental Health Act 1983.

(Department of Health, 2009)

■ A RATIONAL DECISION

To make a competent decision, a degree of rationality is required. It is important that the patient is sufficiently rational to understand and reflect upon their condition in accordance with their own values and belief systems.

- An individual's decision may be influenced by their cultural background and family decision-making practices, wishes and beliefs. Given that individual values and beliefs may vary considerably from person to person, it is possible to understand why the individual's decisions may not always appear rational to others (Department for Constitutional Affairs, 2007, Chapter 3).
- Practitioners must be aware that factors such as fear, anxiety, the effects of medication and pain may affect the patient's ability to consider information and make a rational and competent decision (Department of Health, 2009).

■ WITHDRAWAL OF CONSENT

The adult patient can change their mind at any time – they can withdraw previous consent for treatment or accept information and consent to treatment that was previously declined.

- In instances where the patient withdraws consent, practitioners are advised to ascertain the reason for the withdrawal of consent, discuss the consequences of doing so and attempt to remedy any misconceptions or fears that may be influencing their decision and inhibiting their consent (Department of Health, 2009).

■ SETTLING DISAGREEMENTS

It is in the patient's best interest that disputes or complaints regarding consent to treatment are resolved promptly. Resolution should, in the first instance, be attempted informally via negotiation and discussion with the parties involved. In some instances, where the disagreement cannot be resolved via informal processes, legal advice or a Court declaration may be necessary (British Medical Association, 2008).

Consent and the adult who lacks capacity

■ LASTING POWER OF ATTORNEY

A Lasting Power of Attorney (LPA) is a legal document by which an individual ('the donor') confers authority on another ('the donee', or attorney) to act on their behalf in such a way as to legally bind the person granting that power (Department for Constitutional Affairs, 2007, Chapter 7). An LPA allows a person aged 18 and over to choose someone that they trust to make decisions on their behalf, about things such as their finances or health and wellbeing, at a time in the future when they no longer wish to make those decisions or they may lack the mental capacity to make those decisions themselves. LPAs were introduced with the

Mental Capacity Act in October 2007, replacing Enduring Powers of Attorney (EPA) (Department for Constitutional Affairs, 2007, Chapter 7).

- The Mental Capacity Act 2005 makes it clear that authority conferred by an LPA is subject to the provisions of the Act, and in particular the five statutory key principles (Section 1 of the Act – see Box 1) and the concept of best interests (Section 4 of the Act – see Box 4).
- An LPA can only be made while the individual the attorney will represent still has capacity to make this decision.
- Young people under 18 years of age cannot appoint an attorney/donee.
- There are two types of LPA: Property and Financial Affairs, and Personal Welfare. The LPA document must state what decisions the elected attorney is authorised to make on behalf of the donor. The document must also be registered with the Office of the Public Guardian before its use.
- Individuals may choose to elect a family member or a professional such as a social worker, GP or solicitor to be their attorney/donee providing they have known the donee for two years or more. The donor of an LPA cannot give the donee power to appoint a substitute or successor, but the donor does have the power to appoint a person to replace the donee on the occurrence of certain events (Department for Constitutional Affairs, 2007, Chapter 7).
- All LPAs are regulated by the Office of the Public Guardian (Office of the Public Guardian, 2009).

■ COURT-APPOINTED DEPUTY

When a patient has lost capacity and has not previously appointed an LPA to oversee their affairs, the Court of

Protection may appoint a 'deputy' to act on their behalf (Department for Constitutional Affairs, 2007, Chapter 8).

- Where the Court believes that there is likely to be a need for ongoing decision-making powers on behalf of a person lacking capacity, it may make an appointment under Section 16 (2) of the Mental Capacity Act 2005 to appoint a deputy to act for and make decisions on behalf of the person.
- Two types of deputy can be appointed: one for Health and Welfare and one for Property and Affairs. These are Court appointments and the decision as to who is appointed is based on who the Court believes will act in the patient's best interest where there is nobody willing, or able, to act on the patient's behalf.

(Department for Constitutional Affairs, 2007, Chapter 8)

■ ACTING IN THE BEST INTERESTS OF THE ADULT PATIENT

Decisions about treatment made on behalf of patients who lack capacity should always be made in the patient's best interests, as guided by the Mental Capacity Act 2005 Section 4, and should be the least restrictive to the patient's basic rights and freedoms.

- No one can give consent on behalf of an adult patient who lacks capacity unless they have the authority to do so under an LPA or as a Court-appointed deputy (Department of Health, 2009).
- The patient who lacks capacity to consent may still receive treatment; however, practitioners must be able to justify that all treatment provided is in the patient's best interests as outlined by the Mental Capacity Act 2005. In this way,

the Act offers protection to practitioners from civil and criminal liability when treating adult patients who lack capacity (Department of Health, 2009).

- The Mental Capacity Act 2005 provides a checklist of factors that anyone involved in decision-making must work through when deciding what is in a person's best interests (Box 4).

Box 4
The Mental Capacity Act 2005 Section 4

Best interests

1. In determining for the purposes of this Act what is in a person's best interests, the person making the determination must not make it merely on the basis of—
   a. the person's age or appearance, or
   b. a condition of his, or an aspect of his behaviour, which might lead others to make unjustified assumptions about what might be in his best interests.
2. The person making the determination must consider all the relevant circumstances and, in particular, take the following steps.
3. He must consider—
   a. whether it is likely that the person will at some time have capacity in relation to the matter in question, and
   b. if it appears likely that he will, when that is likely to be.

4. He must, so far as reasonably practicable, permit and encourage the person to participate, or to improve his ability to participate, as fully as possible in any act done for him and any decision affecting him.

5. Where the determination relates to life-sustaining treatment, he must not, in considering whether the treatment is in the best interests of the person concerned, be motivated by a desire to bring about his death.

6. He must consider, so far as is reasonably ascertainable—
   a. the person's past and present wishes and feelings (and, in particular, any relevant written statement made by him when he had capacity),
   b. the beliefs and values that would be likely to influence his decision if he had capacity, and
   c. the other factors that he would be likely to consider if he were able to do so.

7. He must take into account, if it is practicable and appropriate to consult them, the views of—
   a. anyone named by the person as someone to be consulted on the matter in question or on matters of that kind,
   b. anyone engaged in caring for the person or interested in his welfare,
   c. any donee of a Lasting Power of Attorney granted by the person, and
   d. any deputy appointed for the person by the Court, as to what would be in the person's best interests and, in particular, as to the matters mentioned in subsection (6).

8. The duties imposed by subsections (1) to (7) also apply in relation to the exercise of any powers which—
   a. are exercisable under a Lasting Power of Attorney, or
   b. are exercisable by a person under this Act where he reasonably believes that another person lacks capacity.

9. In the case of an act done, or a decision made, by a person other than the Court, there is sufficient compliance with this section if (having complied with the requirements of subsections (1) to (7)) he reasonably believes that what he does or decides is in the best interests of the person concerned.

10. 'Life-sustaining treatment' means treatment which in the view of a person providing health care for the person concerned is necessary to sustain life.

11. 'Relevant circumstances' are those—
    a. of which the person making the determination is aware, and
    b. which it would be reasonable to regard as relevant.

Source: http://www.legislation.gov.uk

- The Mental Capacity Act 2005 stresses that consideration of a patient's 'best interests' goes further than considering only best medical interests and includes considering factors such as: the wishes and beliefs of the patient when competent, their current wishes, their general wellbeing and their spiritual and religious welfare.
- The Mental Capacity Act 2005 reminds practitioners that family, friends and carers close to the individual may be able to provide information on some of the factors to be

considered in the assessment of the patient's best interests. Close family, friends and carers of the patient may be best placed to offer advice on the patient's individual needs and preferences and therefore every effort should be made to include them in the decision-making process.

(Department for Constitutional Affairs, 2007, Chapter 5)

- Consideration of a patient's best interests must not be prejudiced by assumptions about the age, appearance, condition or behaviour of the patient or of persons representing the patient.
- A patient's incapacity to make a decision about their treatment may not be long term. Practitioners need to consider whether the treatment decision can wait until the patient regains the capacity to consent to treatment.

■ ADVANCE DECISIONS AND REFUSAL OF TREATMENT

An advance decision (in the past referred to as a 'living will' or 'advance directive') allows an individual to control the medical treatment they may require at a point in time when they no longer have the capacity to make decisions about that treatment. The individual can decide in advance what types of treatment he or she will or will not accept if they ever lose capacity. Advance decisions are legally binding and must be followed by all healthcare professionals, as long as they meet certain conditions identified in the Mental Capacity Act 2005:

- People under 18 years of age may not make an advance decision.
- At the time of making the decision, the person must have capacity.

- An individual cannot request a particular treatment in an advance decision; only the specific types of treatment the person would *not* wish to be given can be considered.
- The treatments that are being refused must be clearly identified.
- An advance decision need not be in writing to be legally valid, nor are any formal procedures laid down by the Mental Capacity Act 2005. However, if the advance decision is considered by the healthcare provider to apply to 'life-sustaining' treatment, it is recommended that it is made in writing and is witnessed.
- Where it is valid, an advance decision only comes into effect once the individual concerned has lost capacity in relation to the decision(s) it covers.
- The advance decision may be withdrawn at any time by the individual who made it just as long as they have the capacity to do so.

(Department for Health, 2009; Department for Constitutional Affairs, 2007, Chapter 9)

- If a patient becomes incompetent but has clearly indicated in the past, while competent, that they would refuse treatment in certain circumstances (an 'advance refusal') and those circumstances arise, practitioners must abide by that refusal (Department for Constitutional Affairs, 2007, Chapter 9).
- An advance decision cannot be used to give effect to an unlawful act, such as euthanasia, an act which is a deliberate intervention with the express aim of ending life.
- Advance decisions that specifically relate to non-admission to hospital through loss of capacity owing to mental

health reasons, or a clear refusal to be detained, can be overridden and, in these circumstances, the individual can have their liberty removed and be treated without their consent under the Mental Health Act 1986.

(Department for Constitutional Affairs, 2007, Chapter 9)

■ DEPRIVATION OF LIBERTY AND THE ISSUE OF RESTRAINT

The term 'restraint' covers a wide range of actions, which could include confinement and the restriction of movement, e.g. the use of cot sides on a bed, or placing the patient in a locked room. Restraint, defined as the use of or threat of force, may be required to prevent the patient, who lacks capacity, from harm or to persuade the individual to comply with or overcome resistance to treatment considered to be in their best interests (Department for Constitutional Affairs, 2007, Chapter 6).

The use of excessive restraint could lead to a range of civil and criminal penalties against the alleged perpetrator if, in restraining the patient, they are deprived of their liberty.

- The Mental Capacity Act Deprivation of Liberty Safeguards (MCA DOLS 2005), which came into force in England on 1 April 2009, provides a legal framework to prevent the unlawful deprivation of liberty occurring. Primary care trusts (PCTs), local authorities, hospitals and care homes have a statutory responsibility for administering and delivering the MCA DOLS (2005) at a local level.
- Section 5 of the Mental Capacity Act 2005 allows for the use of restraint where it is necessary; however, Section 6 of the Act confirms that there is no protection under Section 5 for actions that result in someone being deprived of their liberty. Deprivations of liberty that do not

result in the person being subject to an application under the Mental Health Act 1983 must be authorised by the Court of Protection to comply with Article 5 of the Human Rights Act 1998.

(Department for Constitutional Affairs, 2007, Chapter 6)

The Mental Capacity Act 2005 identifies three conditions that must be satisfied for the practitioner to be protected from liability when restraining a patient:

1. The patient must lack capacity with regard to the matter in question.
2. The practitioner must reasonably believe that it is necessary to restrain the person who lacks capacity to prevent their harm.
3. Any restraint used must be reasonable and in proportion to the potential harm.

(Royal College of Nursing, 2008)

■ PROVIDING CARE TO PATIENTS WHO LACK CAPACITY

Section 5 of the Mental Capacity Act 2005 provides protection from liability for actions carried out in order to care for an adult who is reasonably believed to lack the capacity to consent for that action. Actions that may be covered include helping the person to maintain everyday activities of living, including personal hygiene, dressing, eating and drinking, and shopping, or treatment such as giving medication and providing nursing care (Department for Constitutional Affairs, 2007, Chapter 6).

- In line with the guiding principles of the Mental Capacity Act 2005 (see Box 1), the activity chosen should be the least restrictive to the person's rights and liberty (Department for Constitutional Affairs, 2007, Chapter 6).

- All activities carried out must serve the best interests of the person.
- Providing care that is respectful and compassionate is crucial.

■ THE PATIENT WITH A MENTAL HEALTH CONDITION

For those individuals for whom detention in hospital is not required, under the terms of the Mental Health Act 1983, the Mental Capacity Act 2005 should be used to guide consent to medical treatment. Just because the patient has a mental health condition does not necessarily mean that they do not have the capacity to make the required treatment decision as determined by the Mental Capacity Act 2005.

However, if a patient is detained under the Mental Health Act 1983, owing to them being a risk to themselves or others, treatment, assessment and decisions must be made in accordance with the Mental Health Act 1983 and not in accordance with the best interests' provisions under the Mental Capacity Act 2005 (Department for Constitutional Affairs, 2007, Chapter 13).

Chapter 13 of the Mental Capacity Act Code of Practice (Department for Constitutional Affairs, 2007) explains when it may be more appropriate for practitioners to refer to the Mental Health Act 1983 instead of the Mental Capacity Act 2005 (Box 5).

- Patients detained under the terms of the Mental Health Act 1983 can be treated for their mental health disorder without their consent even if this goes against an advance decision to refuse that treatment (Department for Constitutional Affairs, 2007, Chapter 13).

Box 5
Department for Constitutional Affairs (DCA) (2007) Mental Capacity Act 2005 Code of Practice

- It is not possible to give the person the care or treatment they need without doing something that might deprive them of their liberty.
- The person needs treatment that cannot be given under the Mental Capacity Act (for example, because the person has made a valid and applicable advance decision to refuse an essential part of treatment).
- The person may need to be restrained in a way that is not allowed under the Mental Capacity Act.
- It is not possible to assess or treat the person safely or effectively without treatment being compulsory (perhaps because the person is expected to regain capacity to consent, but might then refuse to give consent).
- The person lacks capacity to decide on some elements of the treatment but has capacity to refuse a vital part of it – and they have done so, or
- There is some other reason why the person might not get treatment, and they or somebody else might suffer harm as a result.

Source: London: The Stationary Office. Department for Constitutional Affairs http://www.justice.gov.uk/, pp. 225–6.

Children and consent

Unlike adults and young people aged 16 and 17 years of age, children under 16 years of age are presumed to be incompetent, or lack the capacity, to consent to medical treatment unless they prove their competence.

The requirements of a valid consent, as applied to children, are the same as for adults in that to be valid consent must be:

- Given voluntarily.
- Informed by relevant information.
- The child or proxy (someone with parental responsibility) must have the competence or capacity to make the required decision.

(The requirements of a valid consent have been outlined in detail previously.)

■ GILLICK COMPETENCE

To be able to consent to medical treatment, the child must be deemed Gillick-competent/have the capacity to consent. The terms 'competence' and 'capacity' are used interchangeably within the guidance on consent and are taken to mean the same thing. The child must therefore be able to:

- **Understand the purpose of the proposed treatment**, with relevance to the presenting medical issue or condition; namely, the potential benefits, burdens and risks of the proposed treatment and the consequences of not having the treatment.
- Have the **maturity** to understand the wider social, moral and emotional aspects of the decision with relevance to themselves and their family.

- **Fully consider the information and options presented**, which means that the child must be able to retain, use and weigh up the relevant information to inform their decision appropriately.
- **Communicate** their decision clearly to others, so demonstrating their understanding of the information presented and the options available.

(General Medical Council, 2007; Hendrick, 2010)

- The assessment of the child's competence to give consent to treatment is specific to each decision. Each individual decision requires assurance that the child has the competence, understanding and maturity to make that specific decision.
- Naturally some complex treatment decisions will require a higher level of understanding and maturity for the child to be able to assert a competent decision.
- The assessment of Gillick competence reflects the child's developing cognitive ability, maturity and emotional development. Owing to the complexity of some treatment decisions, the child may be able to make some but not all treatment decisions.

(Department of Health, 2009)

- Children with complex health needs and experience of healthcare may, by merit of their past experience, have developed the maturity and understanding to make complex decisions about their treatment beyond that usually expected of a child of their age.
- While a child or young person who is competent can give consent to treatment without their parents' knowledge or additional consent from the parent, it is

considered good practice to involve the child's parents, with the child's permission, in the discussions about treatment, if possible.

(Department of Health, 2009; Hendrick, 2010)

■ THE IMPORTANCE OF INVOLVING CHILDREN IN TREATMENT DECISIONS

Irrespective of the child's level of competence to consent to treatment, it is important that the practitioner makes every effort to respect the child and their developing autonomy by engaging them in discussions about their treatment, listening to their views and interpreting their fears.

- The degree of involvement that each child wishes to have in the decision-making process will vary; some will want to be fully involved and informed while others will defer all decisions to their parents.

■ REFUSAL OF TREATMENT BY A CHILD OR YOUNG PERSON

The competent child under 16 years old, and young person aged 16–17 years of age, can have their refusal to consent to treatment overruled by the Court or a proxy with parental responsibility. Cases of competent refusal of consent by children and young people have been well tested by the Courts, who justify overruling such a decision in cases where the treatment is considered to be life-saving and therefore refusal of treatment would, in all probability, lead to the child's or young person's death or result in severe permanent injury (Department of Health, 2009; Hendrick, 2010).

- Some differences in the law regarding parental responsibility between Scotland and England, Wales and

Northern Ireland exist. One example is that in Scotland the parents cannot overrule the competent refusal of treatment by a young person (General Medical Council, 2007). The practitioner should be cognisant about the difference in application of the law across countries in the UK and should refer to local policies reflecting the law of the land.

- Because of the complexity of the law, in cases involving the overruling of a child's competent refusal of treatment by a person with parental responsibility, when the treatment being refused is considered by practitioners to be in the best interests of the child, practitioners are advised to obtain a decision or declaration from the Court to ensure that treatment in these circumstances is, indeed, lawful (Department of Health, 2009).
- For treatment to be justified as being in the best interests of the child or young person, the benefit of the treatment must outweigh the harm caused by overruling the autonomous decision of the child or young person.

■ THE CHILD WHO IS NOT COMPETENT TO GIVE CONSENT

The Court or a proxy (person with parental responsibility) can give consent to treatment on behalf of a child under 16 years old who is not competent to give consent.

■ PARENTAL RESPONSIBILITY

Parental responsibility is a legal concept that refers to the rights and responsibilities that the majority of parents have regarding their children. A person with parental responsibility has the authority to consent to treatment on behalf of the child under 16 years old (British Medical Association, 2008b). (Box 6 identifies those who have parental responsibility.)

Box 6
People with parental responsibility

- The child's mother.
- The child's father if married to the mother at the time of the birth of the child or thereafter. (In the event of divorce parental responsibility is not lost.)
- Unmarried fathers:

(For children born since 15th April 2002 in Northern Ireland, 1st December 2003 in England and Wales, and 4th May 2006 in Scotland)
   - If recorded (at the time of birth or upon re-registration) on the child's birth certificate jointly with the mother.
- Unmarried fathers whose child's birth was registered before the above dates or unmarried fathers whose child's birth was after the above dates, who are not cited on the child's birth certificate, do not have parental responsibility unless acquired via:
   - Marriage to the mother of the child.
   - A Court-registered responsibility agreement with the mother.
   - A parental responsibility order from the Court.
- Guardians appointed by the Court.
- Adoptive parents.
- Step parents or civil partners can acquire parental responsibility via the Court (agreement or order).

Source: British Medical Association, 2008; Department of Health, 2009; Hendrick, 2010.

- In most cases, consent from one person with parental consent is valid and will suffice even if another person with parental consent disagrees and withholds their consent.
- In some special cases, however, such as non-therapeutic male circumcision, immunisation and experimental treatment, it is not advisable to go ahead with treatment when one person with parental responsibility disagrees with another. Where a person with parental responsibility expresses concern regarding the child's best interests and the benefits of the treatment may be debatable, a decision from the Court should be sought.

(Department of Health, 2009)

- In special cases such as sterilisation for contraceptive purposes, even when those with parental responsibility agree and consent to treatment, guidance from the Court is advised to ensure that treatment is lawful (Department of Health, 2009).
- In some instances, the person with parental responsibility will be under 18 years old themselves. Consent from a person with parental responsibility will be valid only if they themselves have the capacity to give consent.
- Parental responsibility is not an absolute right. The Court can overrule the decision of the person with parental responsibility if their decision is not deemed to be in the best interests of the child.
- If the person with parental responsibility is not considered to be acting in the best interests of the child, then their consent cannot be relied upon. In such instances, practitioners must follow local safeguarding

policies to secure the safety and protection of the child, and legal advice may be necessary to inform treatment decisions.

(Department of Health, 2009)

■ THE BEST INTERESTS OR WELFARE PRINCIPLE

Any decision made on behalf of a child should be done with the child's best interests or welfare in mind (the terms 'best interests' and 'welfare' are used interchangeably). Both the Children Act 1989 Section 1 and case law define the factors that need to be considered when making a decision in the best interests of the child (Box 7).

Box 7
Consideration of the best interests of the child

Assessment of best interests includes consideration of, but should not be limited to, medical factors and should include:

- Emotional, psychological and social factors.
- The likely impact of the decision on the child.
- Actual and likely harm and risk to the child.
- The child's age, sex, background and any other characteristics considered to inform the decision.
- The wishes and feelings of the child, including cultural and religious beliefs.
- The views of the parents, those close to the child and healthcare practitioners involved with the child.

Source: The Children Act 1989 Section 1; Hendrick, 2010.

■ DISAGREEMENTS

Occasionally there may be disagreements between parents and practitioners regarding the consideration of the best interests of the child. If such disagreements cannot be resolved by negotiation and communication, then legal advice should be sought and a decision from the Court may be required to guide treatment.

Young people and consent

■ CAPACITY

Just like adults, young people aged 16–17 years are presumed competent to make a decision about medical treatment unless proven to lack capacity. The Mental Capacity Act 2005 guides the assessment of capacity for a young person aged 16–17 years (see Boxes 2 and 3).

If a young person of 16–17 years is considered to lack capacity in line with Section 2 (1) of the Mental Capacity Act 2005 (see Box 2), then the Act applies for the young person just as it does for the adult of 18 years and over. If, however, the young person cannot make the required decision because they are 'overwhelmed' by it, this is not covered by the Mental Capacity Act 2005, and in this instance the Act will not apply. Instead, common law principles should be used to assess the legality of treatment, and guidance relating to parental responsibility (Box 6) and best interests (Box 7) will apply (Department of Health, 2009; Department for Constitutional Affairs, 2007, Chapter 12).

■ PARTS OF THE MENTAL CAPACITY ACT 2005 THAT DO NOT APPLY TO YOUNG PEOPLE OF 16–17 YEARS

Young people under 18 years of age cannot do the following:

- Make an LPA.
- Make an advance decision to refuse treatment.
- Make a will.

(Department for Constitutional Affairs, 2007, Chapter 12)

- Under the terms of the Mental Capacity Act 2005, the young person aged 16–17 years cannot consent to any treatments that are not of direct benefit to their health, such as organ donation and participation in research. Instead, to give their consent to such treatments, the young person would have to be deemed Gillick-competent (Department of Health, 2009).

References

Brazier, M. and Cave, E. (2007) *Medicine, Patients and The Law*. London: Penguin Books.

Bristol Royal Infirmary Inquiry (Kennedy Report) (2001) *Learning from Bristol: The Report of the Public Inquiry into Children's Heart Surgery at the Bristol Royal Infirmary 1984–1995*. Command Paper: CM 5207. London: The Stationery Office.

British Medical Association (BMA) (2008) *Parental Responsibility: Guidance from the British Medical Association*. London: British Medical Association.

British Medical Association (BMA) (2008a) *Mental Capacity Act Toolkit*. London: British Medical Association.

British Medical Association (BMA) (2008b) *Parental Responsibility: Guidance from the British Medical Association.* London: British Medical Association.

Department for Constitutional Affairs (DCA) (2007) *Mental Capacity Act 2005 Code of Practice.* London: The Stationery Office.

Department of Health (DH) (2009) *Reference Guide to Consent for Examination or Treatment* (2nd edn). London: Department of Health.

Department of Health (DH) (2012) *Compassion in Practice: Nursing, Midwifery and Care Staff: Our Vision and Strategy.* Leeds: Department of Health.

Dimond, B. (2011) *Legal Aspects of Nursing* (6th edn). Essex: Pearson Education Limited.

General Medical Council (GMC) (2007) *0–18 Years: Guidance for all Doctors.* London: General Medical Council.

General Medical Council (GMC) (2008) *Consent: Patients and Doctors Making Decisions Together.* London: General Medical Council.

Health and Care Professions Council (HCPC) (2012) *Your Duties as a Registrant: Standards of Conduct, Performance and Ethics.* London: Health and Care Professions Council.

Hendrick, J. (2010) *Law and Ethics in Children's Nursing.* West Sussex: Wiley-Blackwell.

Nursing and Midwifery Council (NMC) (2008) *The Code: Standards of Conduct, Performance and Ethics for Nurses and Midwives.* London: Nursing and Midwifery Council.

Office of the Public Guardian (2009) *The Mental Capacity Act – Making Decisions: A Guide for Family, Friends and Other Unpaid Carers* (OPG602) (4th edn). London: Office of the Public Guardian.

Royal College of Nursing (RCN) (2008) *Let's Talk about Restraint: Rights, Risks and Responsibility*. London: Royal College of Nursing.

Useful websites

British Medical Association:
http://bma.org.uk/

Department for Constitutional Affairs:
http://www.justice.gov.uk/

Department of Health:
http://www.dh.gov.uk/en/index.htm

General Medical Council:
http://www.gmc-uk.org/

Health and Care Professions Council:
http://www.hpc-uk.org/

Mental Health Organisation:
http://www.mentalhealth.org.uk/

Nursing and Midwifery Council:
http://www.nmc-uk.org/

Royal College of Paediatrics and Child Health:
http://www.rcpch.ac.uk/

The Children Act 1989:
http://www.legislation.gov.uk/ukpga/1989 ÷ 41/ introduction

The Human Rights Act 1998:
http://www.legislation.gov.uk/ukpga/1998/42/contents

The Mental Health Act 1983:
http://www.legislation.gov.uk/ukpga/1983/20/contents

The Mental Capacity Act 2005:
http://www.legislation.gov.uk/ukpga/2005/9/contents

T - #0269 - 071024 - C0 - 120/80/2 - SB - 9780273775171 - Gloss Laminatic